WELLNESS
MIND BODY MOTION

YOGA

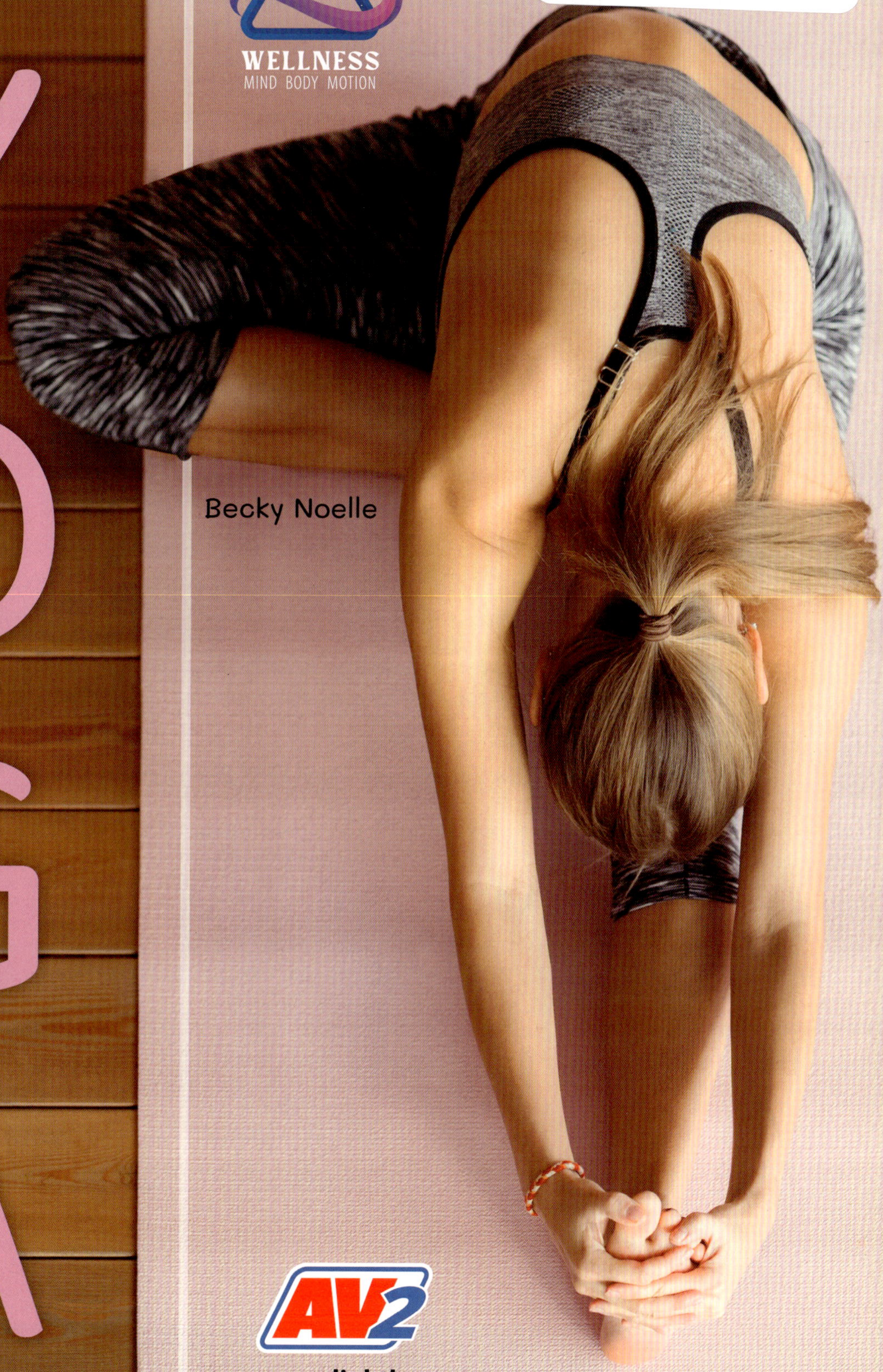

Becky Noelle

AV2
www.openlightbox.com

AV2

Step 1
Go to **www.openlightbox.com**

Step 2
Enter this unique code
RIVUM4RWS

Step 3
Explore your interactive eBook!

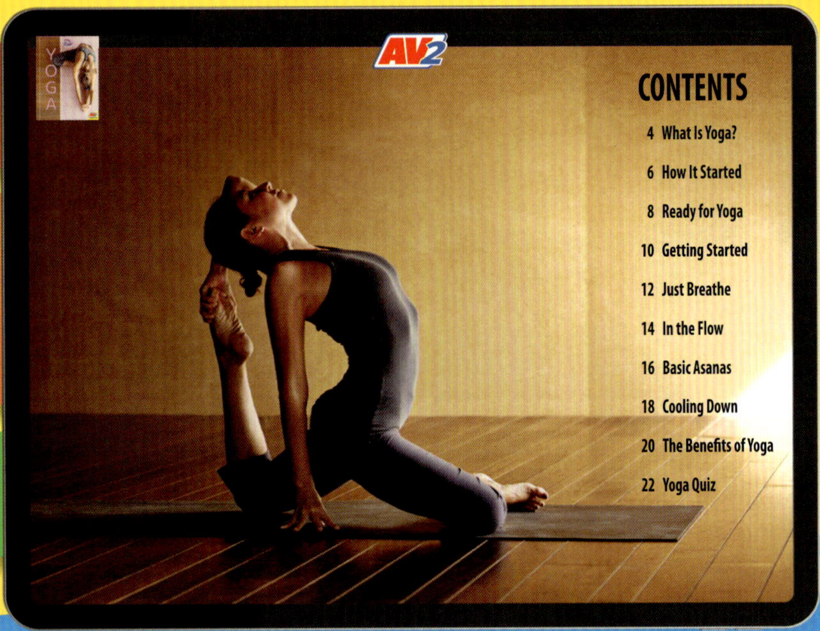

AV2 is optimized for use on any device

Your interactive eBook comes with...

Contents
Browse a live contents page to easily navigate through resources

Audio
Listen to sections of the book read aloud

Videos
Watch informative video clips

Weblinks
Gain additional information for research

Slideshows
View images and captions

Try This!
Complete activities and hands-on experiments

Key Words
Study vocabulary, and complete a matching word activity

Quizzes
Test your knowledge

Share
Share titles within your Learning Management System (LMS) or Library Circulation System

Citation
Create bibliographical references following the Chicago Manual of Style

This title is part of our AV2 digital subscription

1-Year 3–8 Subscription
ISBN 978-1-7911-3306-1

Access hundreds of AV2 titles with our digital subscription.
Sign up for a FREE trial at **www.openlightbox.com/trial**

WELLNESS
MIND BODY MOTION

YOGA

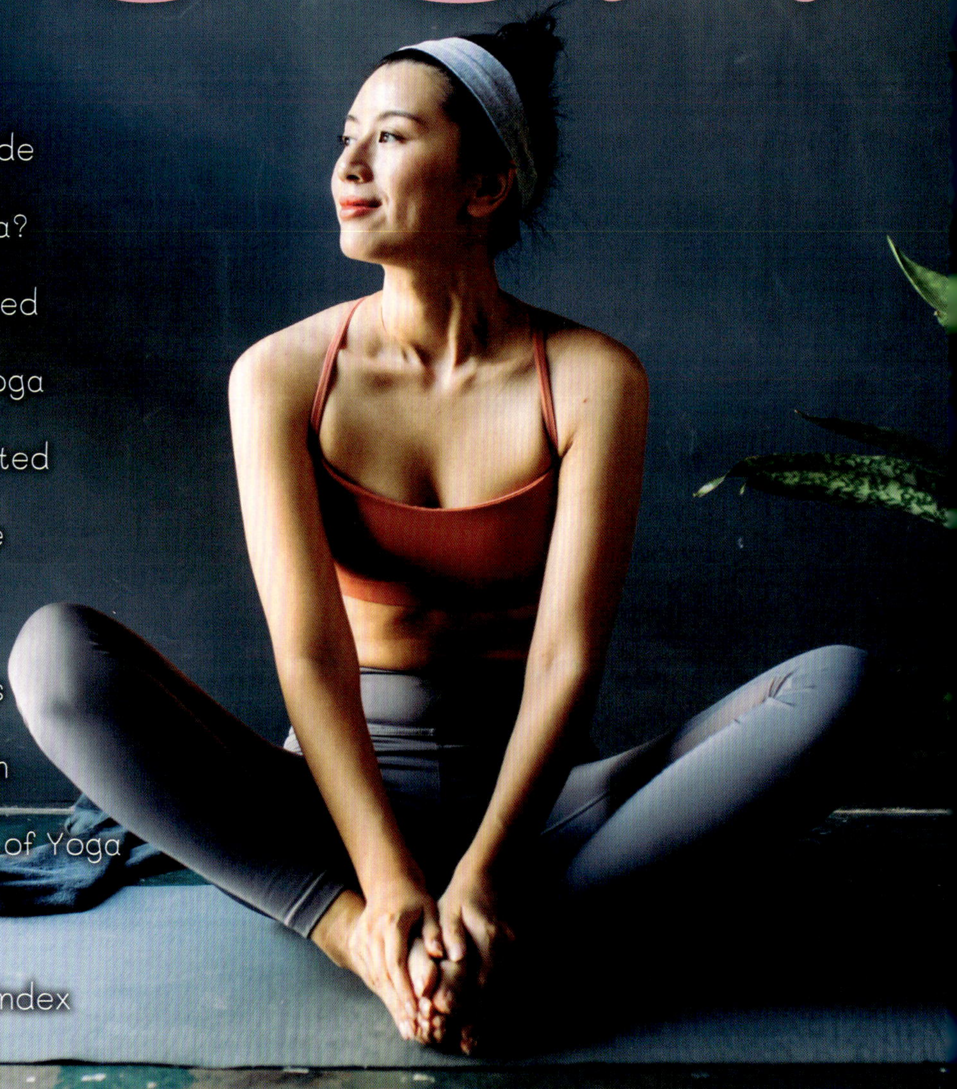

What Is Yoga?

Yoga is a popular activity that people from all around the world do to stay calm and healthy. It started in India as a way for people to connect their mind, body, and spirit. *Yoga* is a **Sanskrit** word that means "to connect."

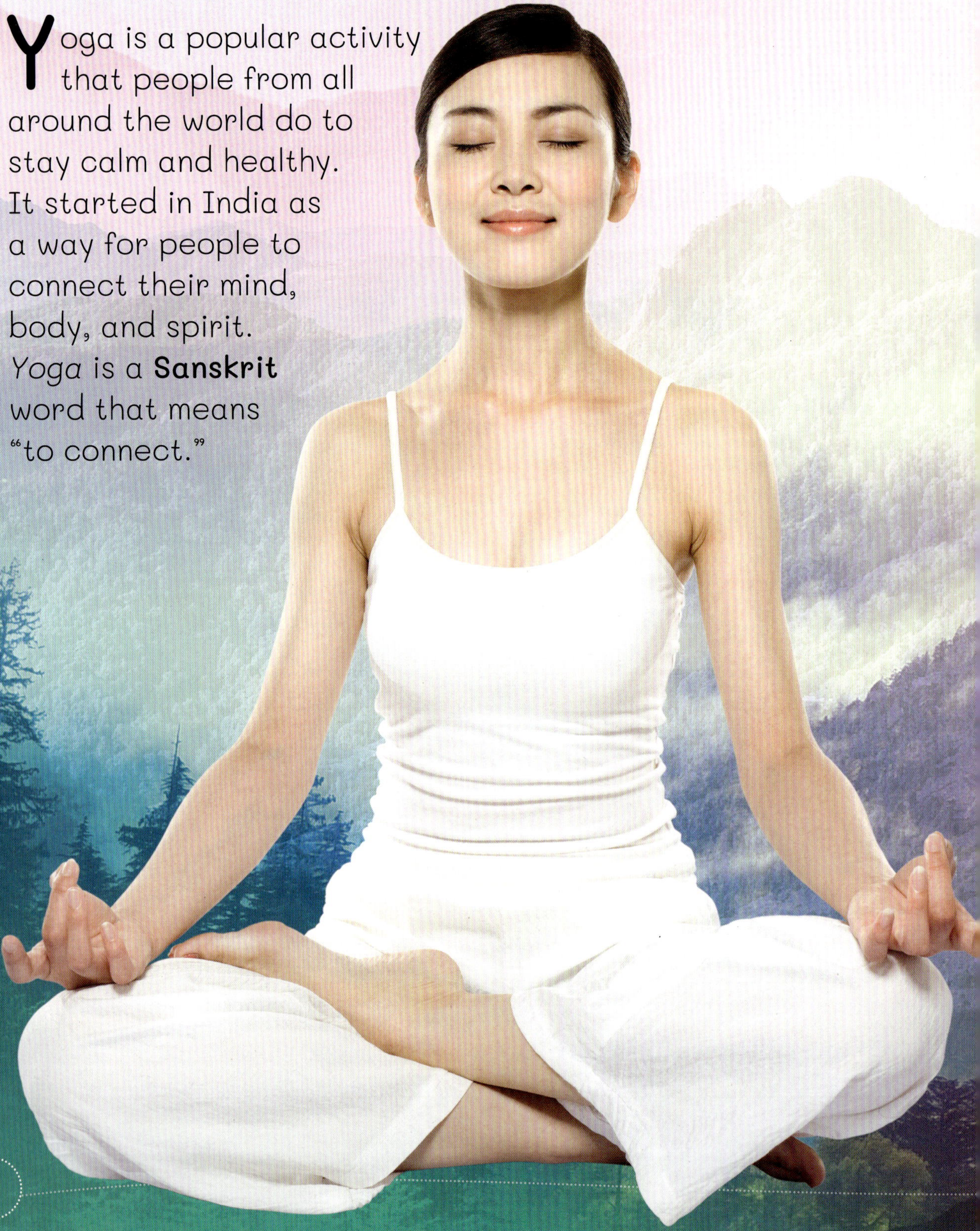

Yoga is centered around breathing exercises, body **poses**, and **meditation**. Breathing exercises, called *pranayama*, allow people to focus on their breath, and how it moves in and out of their body. Body poses, or *asanas*, stretch and strengthen different parts of the body. Meditation helps people calm their minds and connect with their spirits.

Yoga is known for its gentle movement. Almost anyone can **practice** it. Yoga is a great way to calm the mind and keep the body healthy.

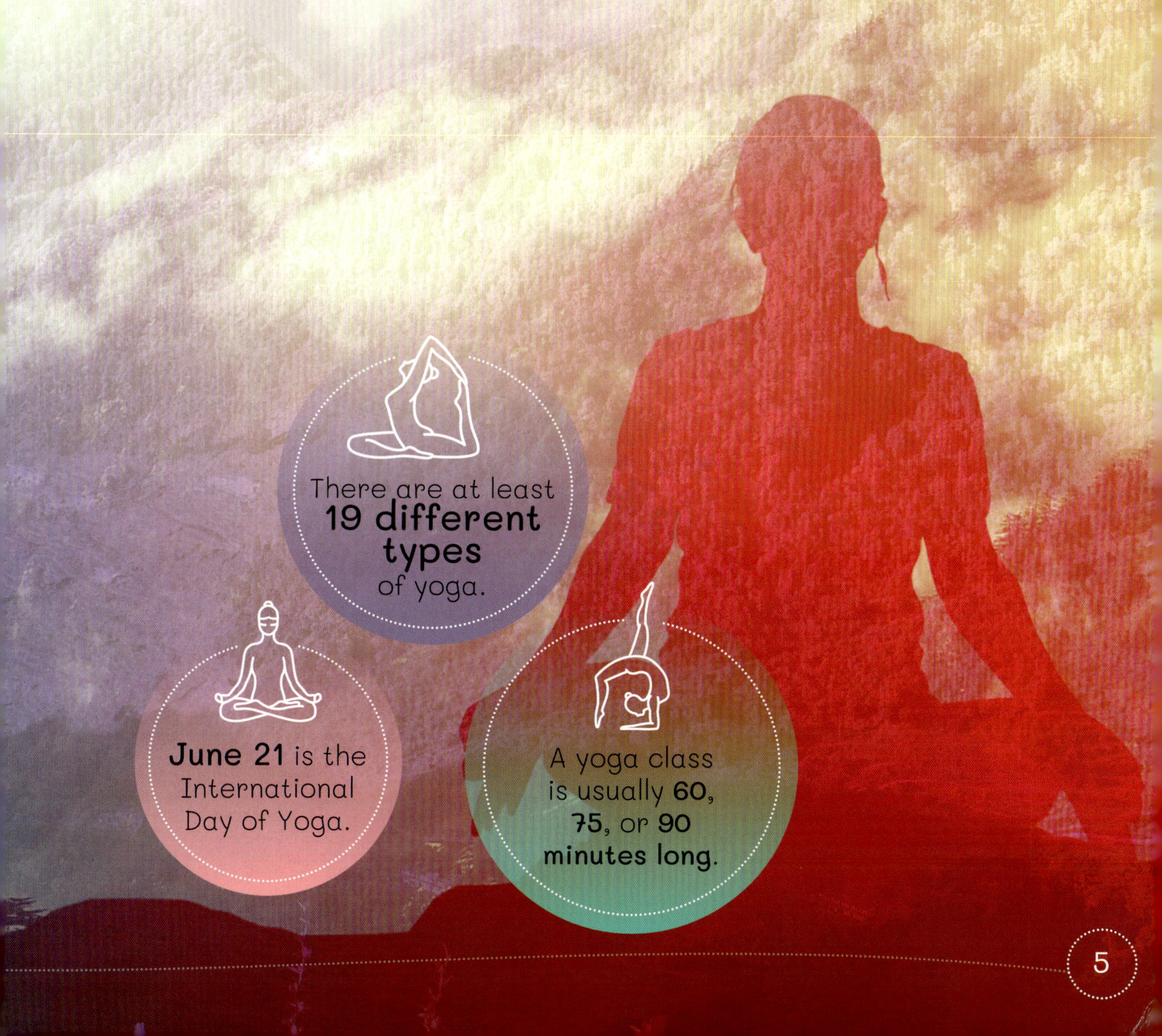

There are at least **19 different types** of yoga.

June 21 is the International Day of Yoga.

A yoga class is usually **60, 75, or 90 minutes long.**

How It Started

Yoga has connections to the Hindu and Buddhist religions. It has been practiced for thousands of years. Many people say that Shiva, a Hindu god, was the first **yogi**. The Buddha, the founder of Buddhism, created his own yoga teachings much later.

The *Yoga Sutras* is an important book about yoga. It is believed to have been written by a man named Maharishi Patañjali more than 1,500 years ago. The sutras explain what yoga is and how it can be practiced.

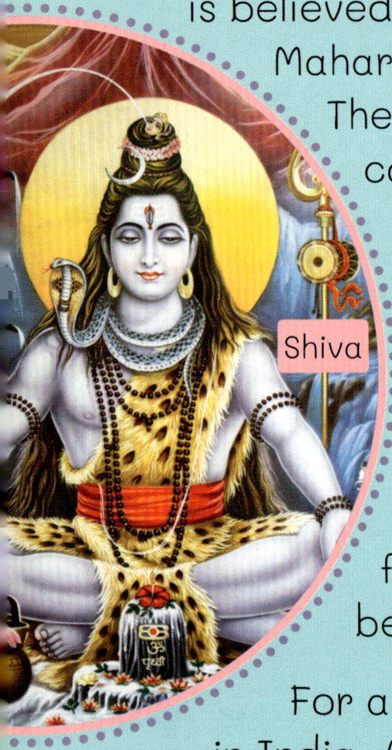
Shiva

Before the 20th century, yoga had very few standing poses. This changed in the 1920s, when teachers added movements from wrestling and gymnastics into their classes. One such teacher was Tirumalai Krishnamacharya, who was known as the father of modern yoga. After this, yoga began to be seen as a form of exercise.

For a long time, yoga was mostly practiced in India. A European woman known as Indra Devi went to India to study with Krishnamacharya. She later moved to the United States, where she taught others what she had learned. Yoga became popular there. Over time, it spread to other parts of the world. Today, about 300 million people practice yoga worldwide.

Timeline

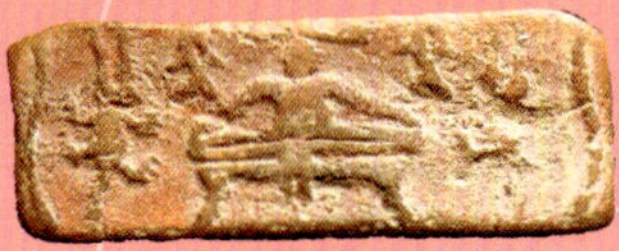

2700 BC Artwork that shows people doing yoga is created in the Indus Valley in India.

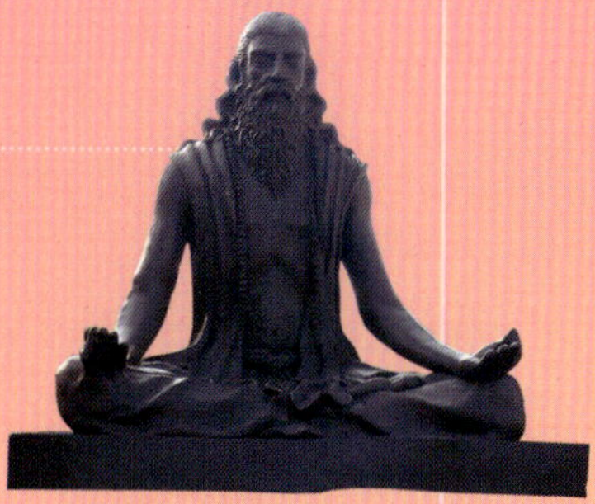

400 AD Maharishi Patañjali writes the *Yoga Sutras*.

1851 Nobin Chunder Paul, an Indian scientist, writes about the health benefits of yoga.

1920s With the addition of standing poses, yoga begins to be seen as a form of exercise.

1947 Indra Devi moves to the United States and teaches yoga to Hollywood stars.

2020 An international survey shows yoga to be the most popular digital workout of 2020.

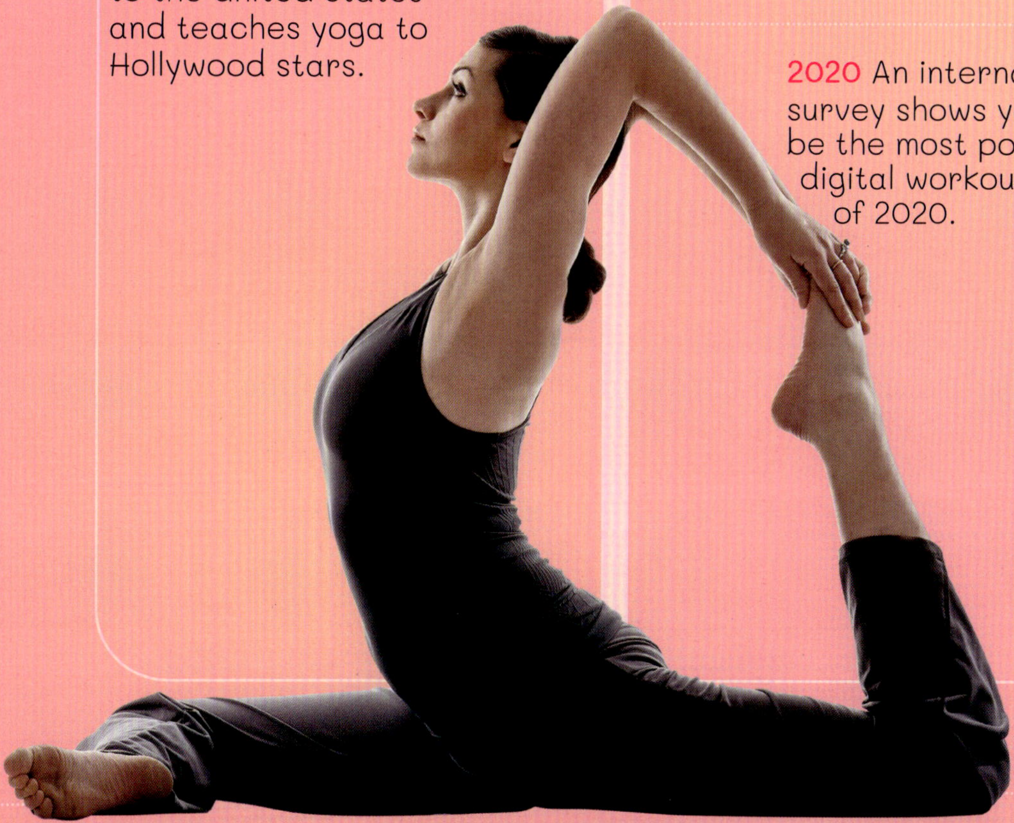

Ready for Yoga

Yoga can be done almost anywhere and anytime. What is important is that the person doing yoga is comfortable. Most people prefer to wear tight, stretchy clothes when doing yoga. Tight clothes stay in place when the body is moving. Wearing stretchy clothes makes it easier to move.

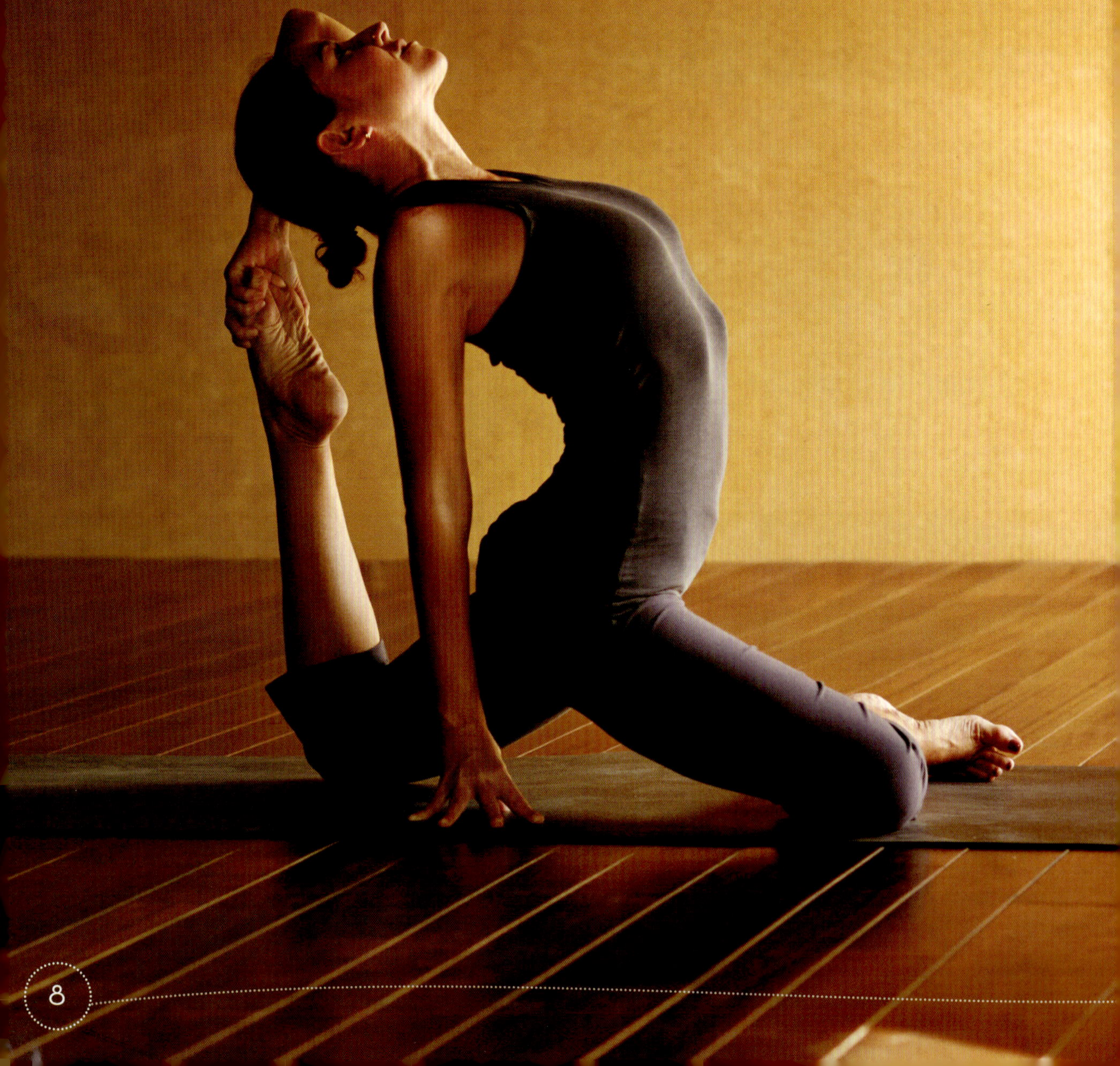

Equipment

Yoga does not require much equipment. However, there are some items that can help people stay safe and comfortable.

Mat

Yoga mats provide a cushion between the person and the floor's surface. This makes sitting and kneeling more comfortable. The mat also prevents slipping by keeping the feet in place during standing poses.

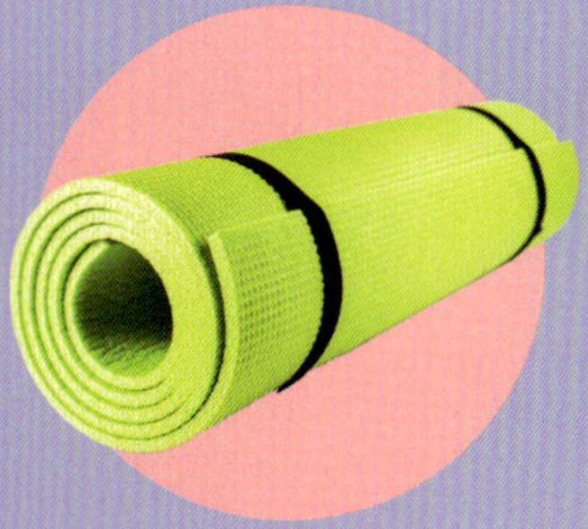

Blocks

Yoga blocks are used to make poses easier. Sometimes, people may not be able to reach their hands to the floor during a pose. They can lean on a block instead. Yoga blocks can be set at three different heights. This allows people to reach as far as needed to hold a pose.

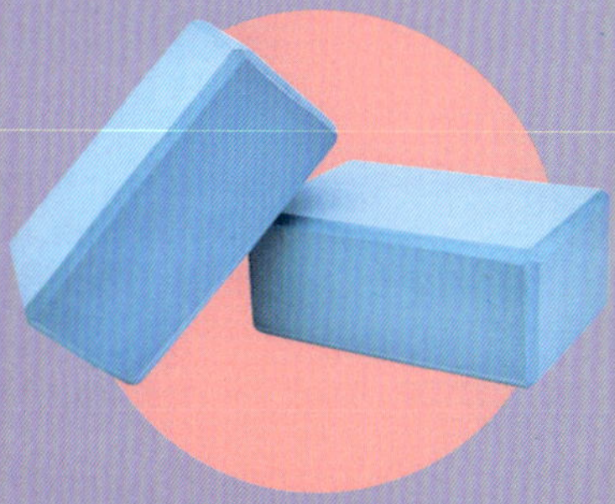

Strap

Yoga straps help people stretch. Some people might not be able to stretch far enough to complete a pose. A strap can help them hold onto their feet when stretching out their legs. It can also help them link their hands behind their back.

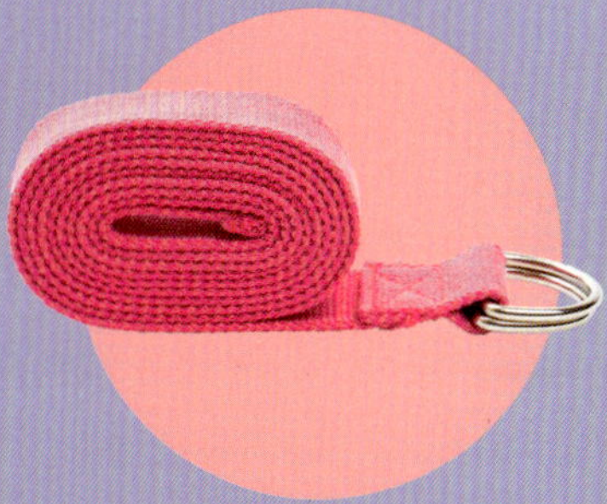

Water Bottle

Like any exercise, yoga can make people sweat. It is important to stay **hydrated** while doing yoga. Drinking water is the best way to stay hydrated. Having a full water bottle nearby is essential.

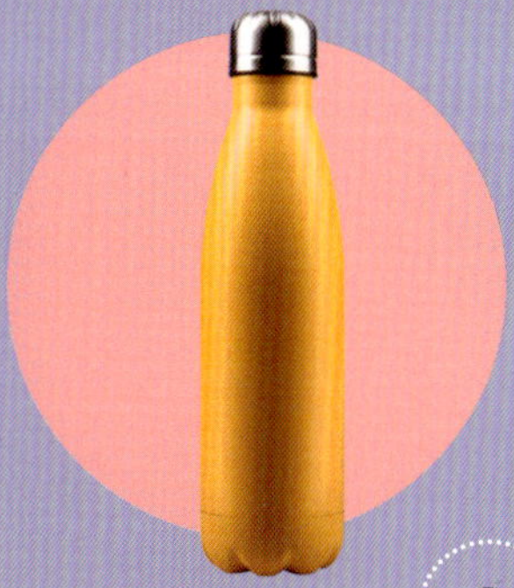

Getting Started

The beginning of a yoga class is a time to clear the mind of worries and focus on how the body feels. To do this, the yoga teacher, or guru, often takes students through a few minutes of pranayama. The guru might ask the students to think about their goals for the class. This is called setting an **intention**. Once their thoughts and breathing have settled, the class will begin to do poses. Each pose has its own name.

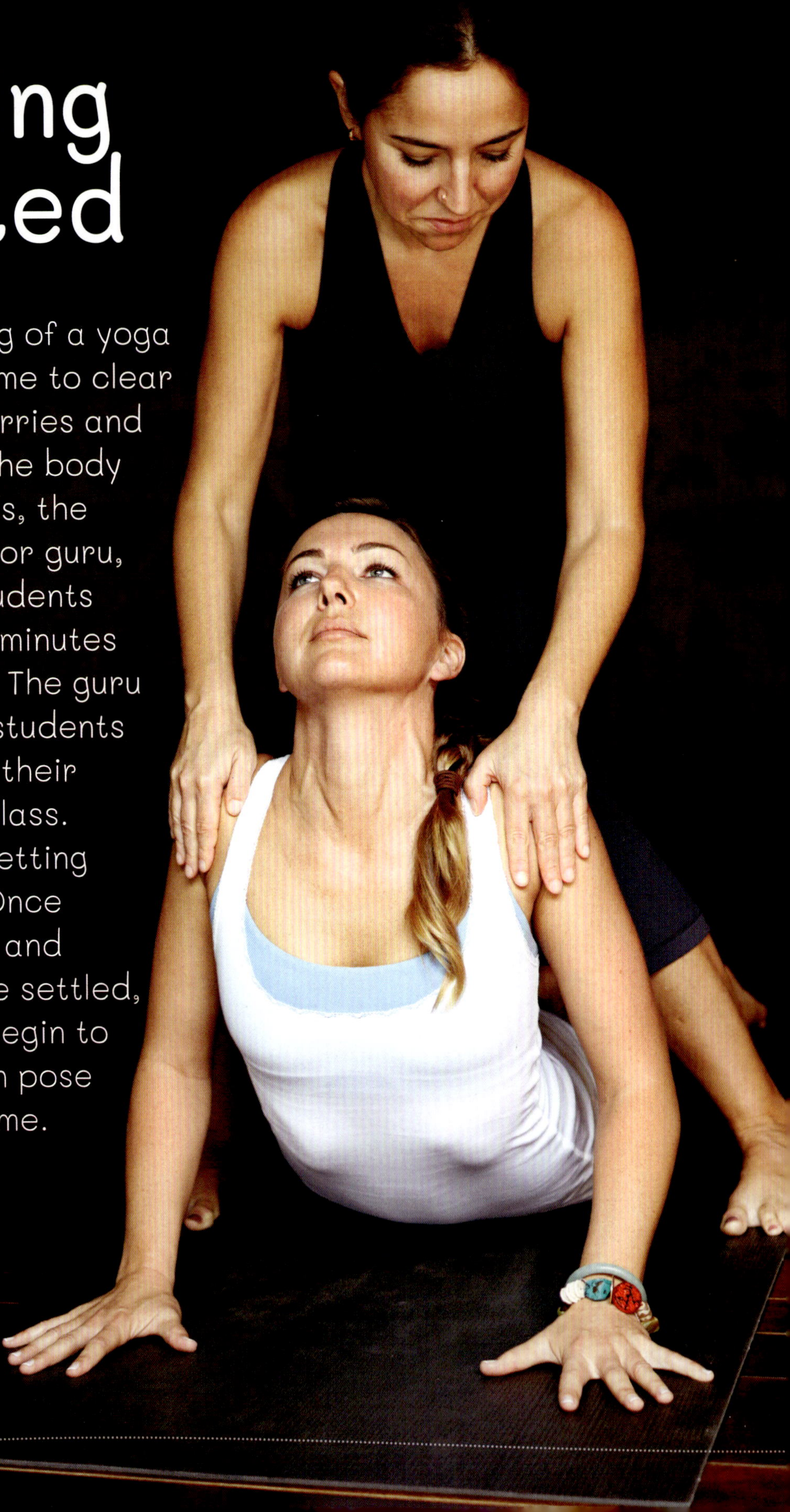

To stay safe during a yoga class, students must slowly warm up their muscles. Difficult poses should be saved for the middle or end of a class. At the start of a class, students will do gentle stretches and easier poses. These stretches and poses will use the same muscles as the more difficult poses performed later in the class.

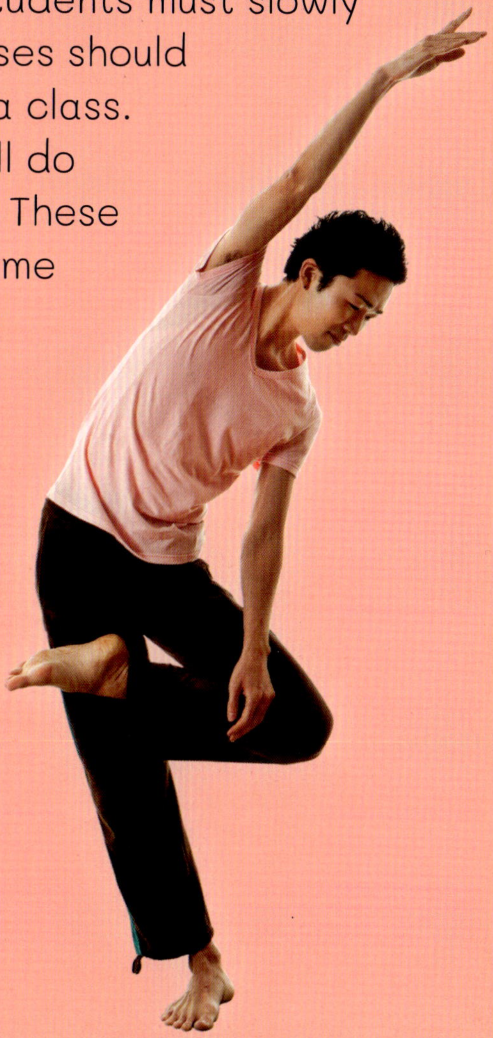

During a yoga class, the guru tells the students what poses and breathing exercises to do. The guru might demonstrate the poses or give tips on how to do a pose well. Gurus are trained in yoga and know how to make sure everyone is doing the poses safely. They can help students check their **alignment**, so they do not get hurt during a pose.

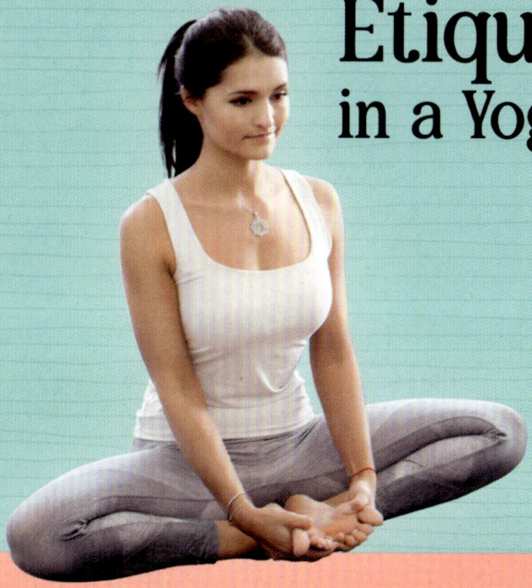

Etiquette in a Yoga Class

A yoga class is a time for quiet and calm. To show respect to the other students, do not make loud noises or talk during a class. Electronic devices should be turned off. Focus on what the guru tells you to do, and do your best to try each pose without distracting others.

Just Breathe

You can practice pranayama at home. It will help you focus on different ways of breathing. For example, belly breathing helps you focus on taking big, deep breaths, filling your belly and chest with air. **Ratio** breathing focuses on how long you inhale and exhale. When people feel **stressed**, they take quick, shallow breaths. By paying attention to your breath, you can start to notice how it feels to take slow, full breaths.

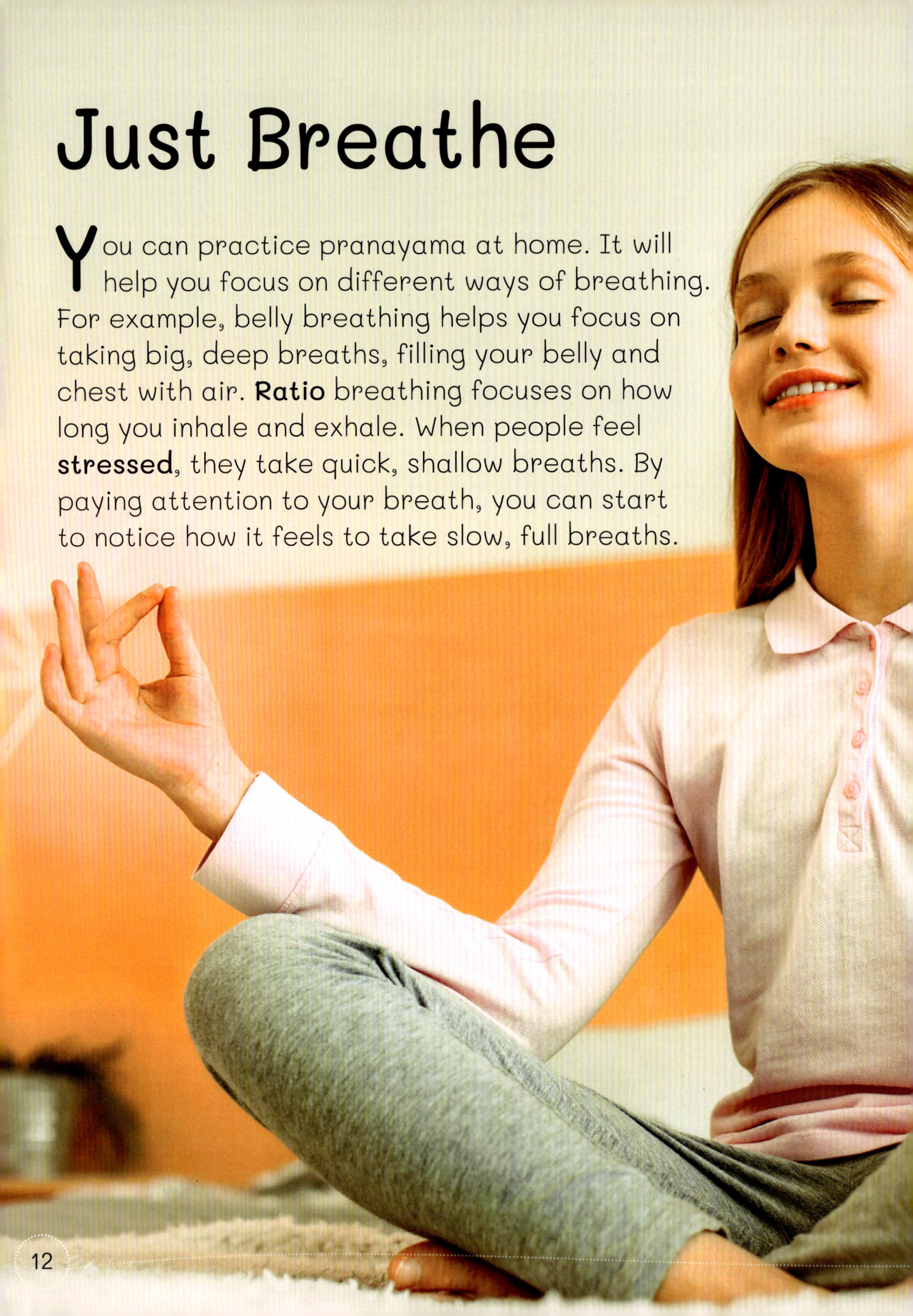

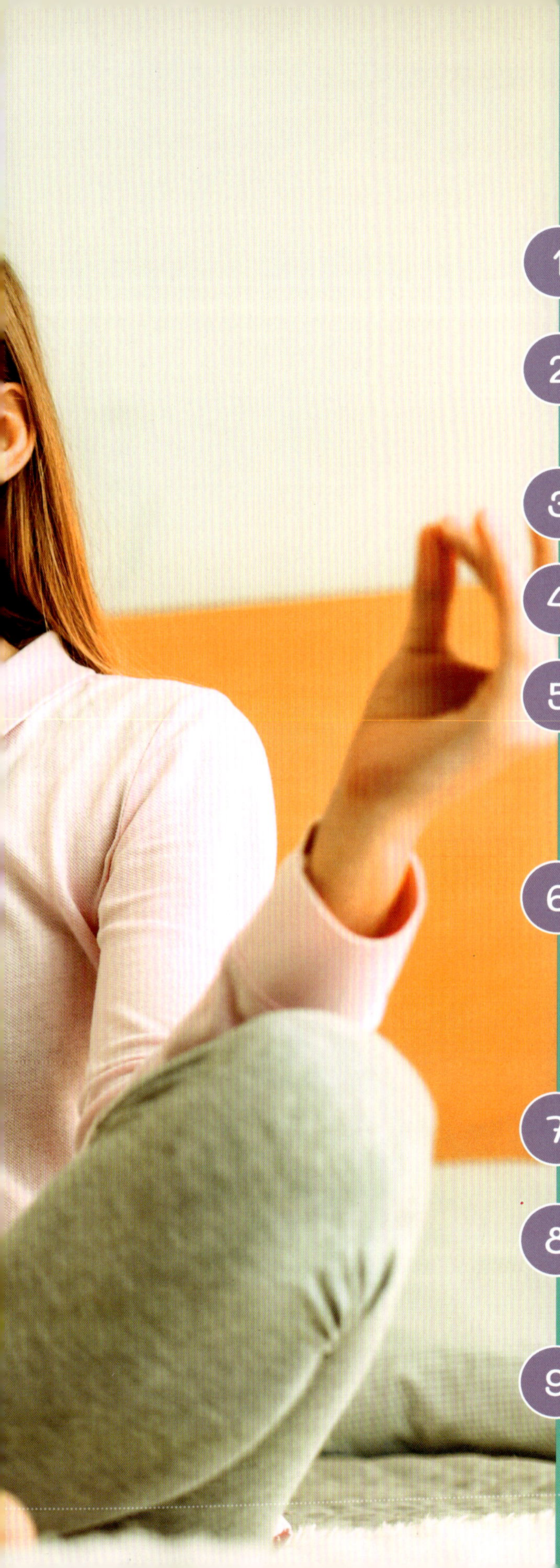

Try ratio breathing for yourself.

1. Sit cross-legged on a yoga mat or the floor.
2. Straighten your back. Imagine a string is pulling your head up toward the ceiling.
3. Relax your shoulders, and rest your hands gently on your knees.
4. Close your eyes.
5. Breathe in through your nose while you count to four. Keep breathing in until you get to four. Remember to fill up your belly and your chest as you breathe in.
6. Slowly breathe out while you count to four again. Keep breathing out until you get to four. Think about pushing all the air out of your belly and then your chest as you breathe out.
7. Continue this pattern until you feel comfortable and calm.
8. Try breathing in for four counts and out for six or breathing in for five counts and out for five.
9. Next time you feel stressed, try ratio breathing and see how calm you can get.

In the Flow

A yoga class can progress in different ways. It all depends on the type of yoga being practiced. Some classes focus on holding poses. Others may require more movement.

During a *yin* yoga class, students will hold their poses for anywhere from three to five minutes. It can be difficult to keep a clear mind during a long pose. Students use their breath to stay focused.

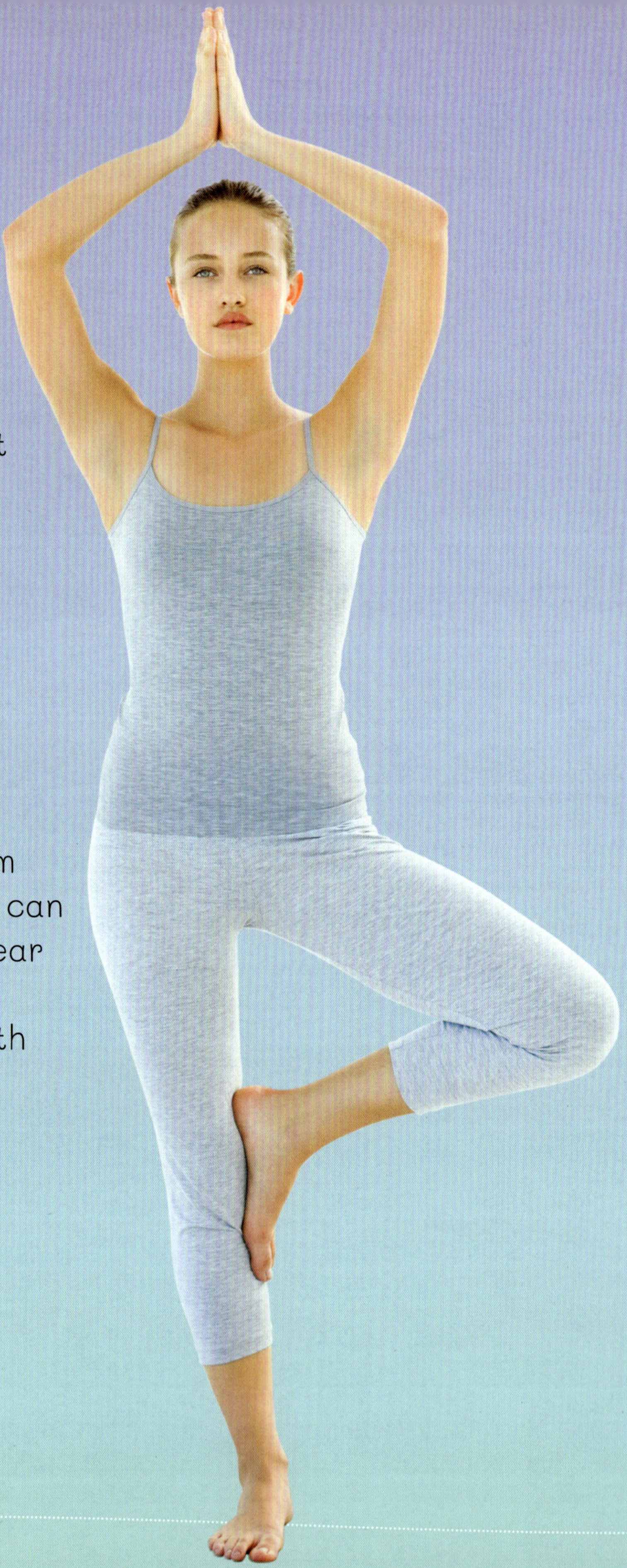

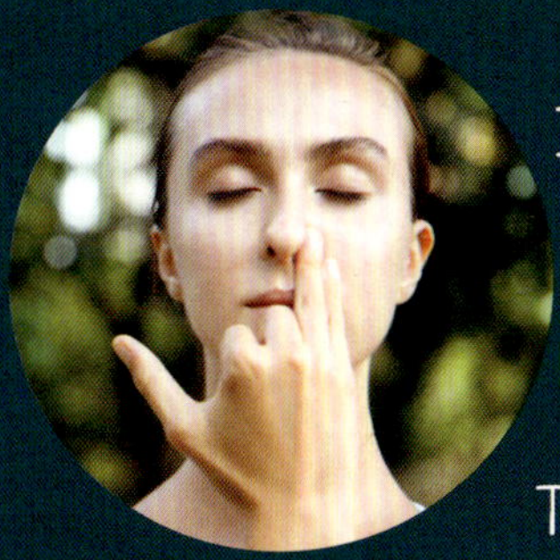

In a *vinyasa* yoga class, students begin to flow from one pose to the next. They may start in mountain pose, by standing straight and tall with their feet together. They then begin moving from standing poses to lower poses. A vinyasa class may gradually build up to more difficult poses.

During a *hatha* class, students practice pranayama while they hold poses. They might cover one nostril as they breathe in and out, or make specific sounds as they breathe. These **techniques** help them notice their breath and slow it down.

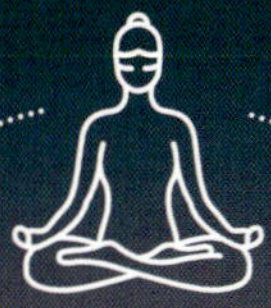

In 2017, Jagadeesan Settu, from India, completed the **longest yoga marathon**. It lasted for **138 hours and 14 minutes.**

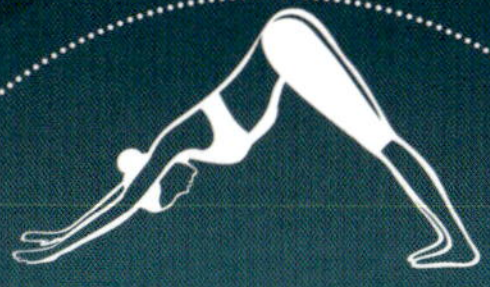

Kiki Flynn holds the world record for the **longest** downward dog pose. She did the pose for **60 minutes and 18 seconds**.

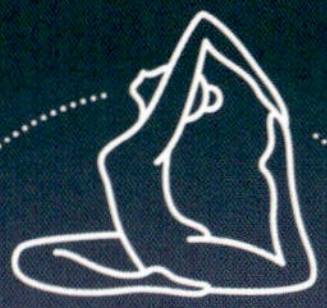

Yoga has **84** key poses.

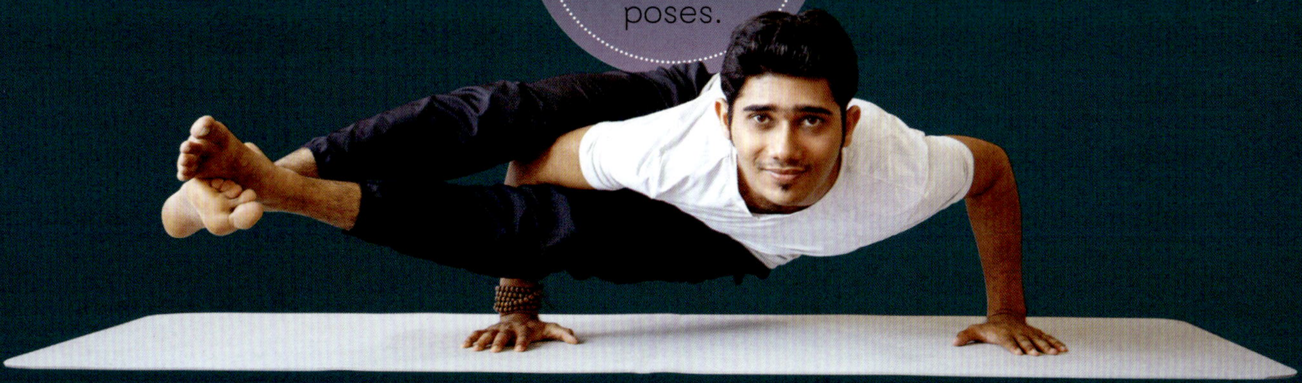

Basic Asanas

There are several basic poses that people learn when starting to practice yoga. These asanas help new students become comfortable with their bodies and gain confidence using them. These three asanas are some of the most popular. To get started, practice them with an adult for the first few times.

Downward Dog

In a downward dog pose, the body makes an upside-down V shape, much like a stretching dog does.

1. Get onto your hands and knees on the yoga mat.
2. Curl your toes under so they are touching the mat.
3. Push back through your hands to lift your hips up into the air.
4. Keep your hands flat on the mat and your arms straight.
5. Push your chest toward your knees. Your knees can be bent or straight.
6. Gently reach your heels toward the mat only as far as they will go.

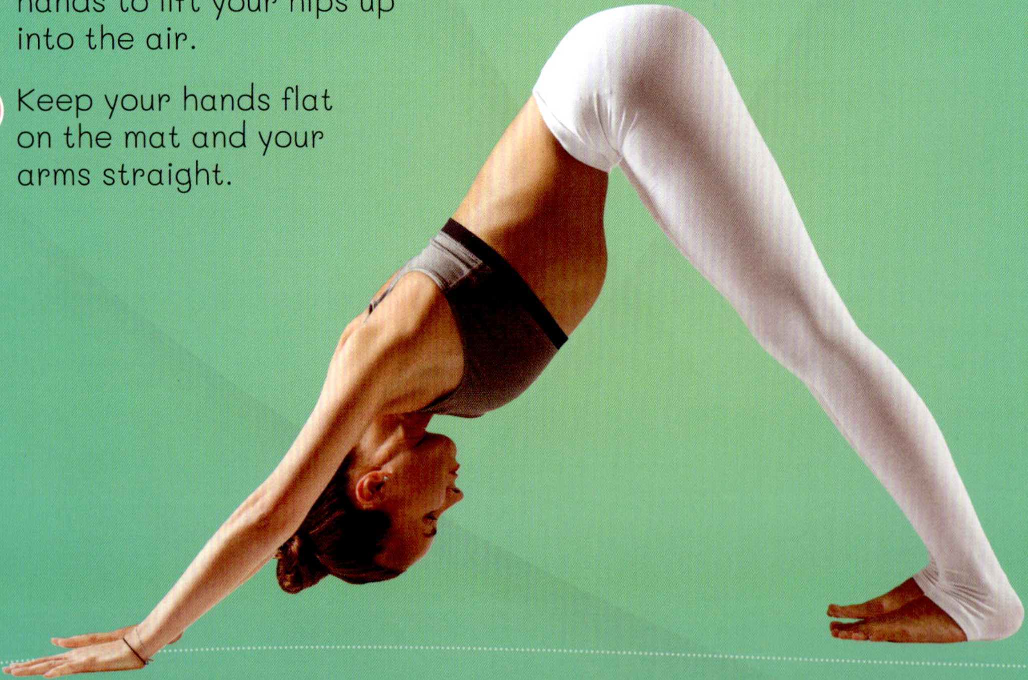

Cobra

A cobra pose is a deep back bend that makes you look like a snake with its head up.

1. Lie on your belly on the yoga mat with the tops of your feet and forehead touching the mat.
2. Put your hands flat on the mat under your shoulders.
3. Keep your elbows close to your body.
4. Use your arm and back muscles to gently lift your head and chest up.
5. Stop when you feel a stretch in your back. Do not push too far up to avoid hurting your back.

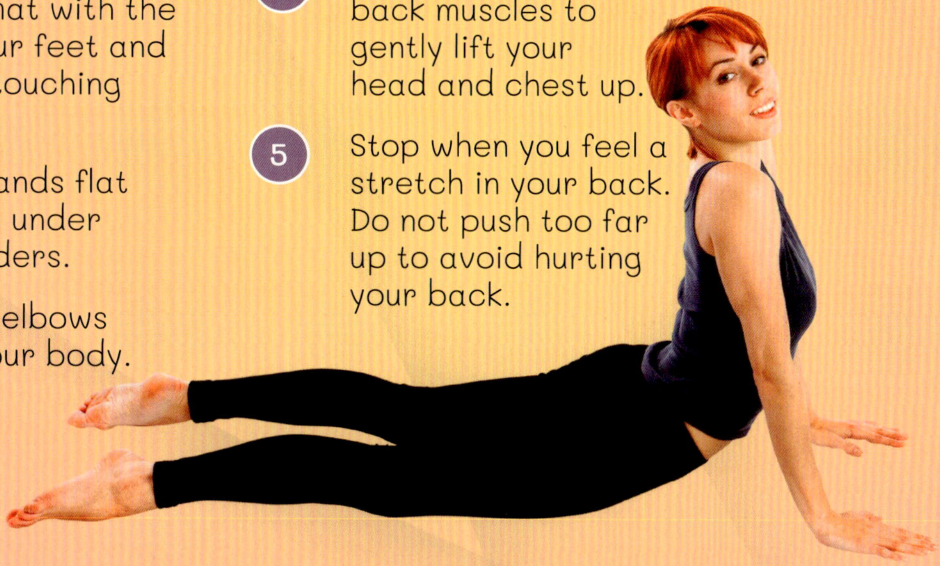

Warrior II

Yoga has five warrior poses. They help to strengthen and stretch your leg muscles.

1. To begin warrior II, stand with your legs close together and your toes pointing forward.
2. Step back with one leg.
3. Turn your back toes so they are facing to the side.
4. Bend your front knee. Keep your back leg straight.
5. Stretch your arms out straight from your sides with your palms facing the floor.
6. Look forward in the direction of your bent knee.

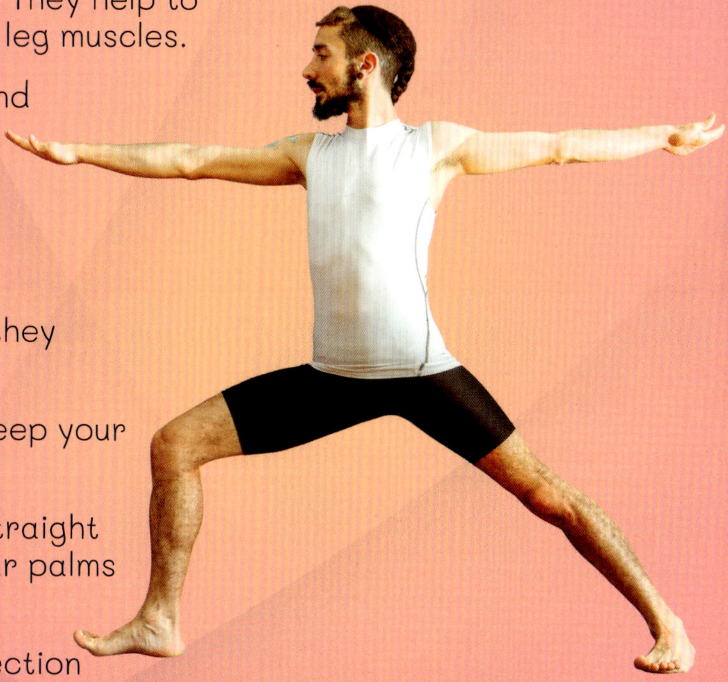

Cooling Down

Before finishing a yoga session, it is important to cool down. Poses near the end of class are usually done sitting or lying down. Students stretch out the muscles that were used most during class. This might include leg and hip stretches or twists.

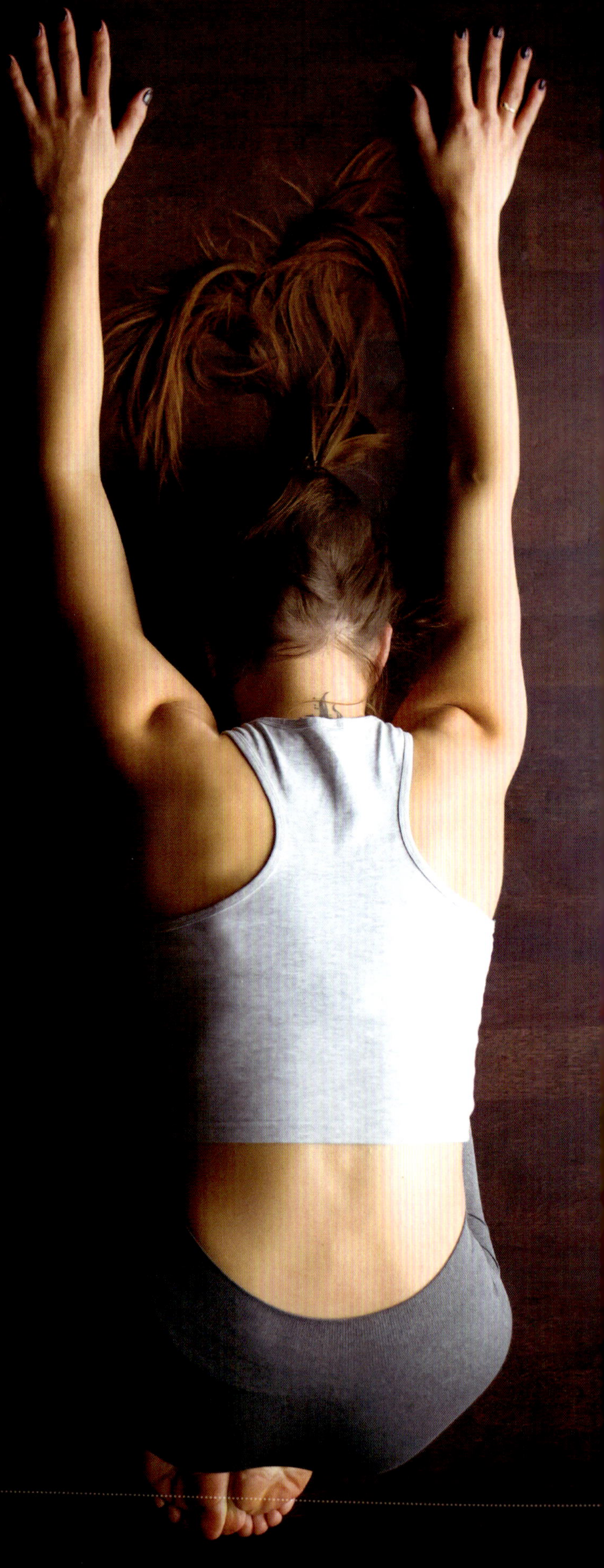

At the very end of a yoga class, everyone performs *savasana*. For this pose, people lie flat on their backs with their legs and arms stretched out, palms facing up. They close their eyes and pay attention to how their body feels. During savasana, everyone lets their body completely relax. This pause at the end of class gives them time to notice the effects that the class has had on their bodies.

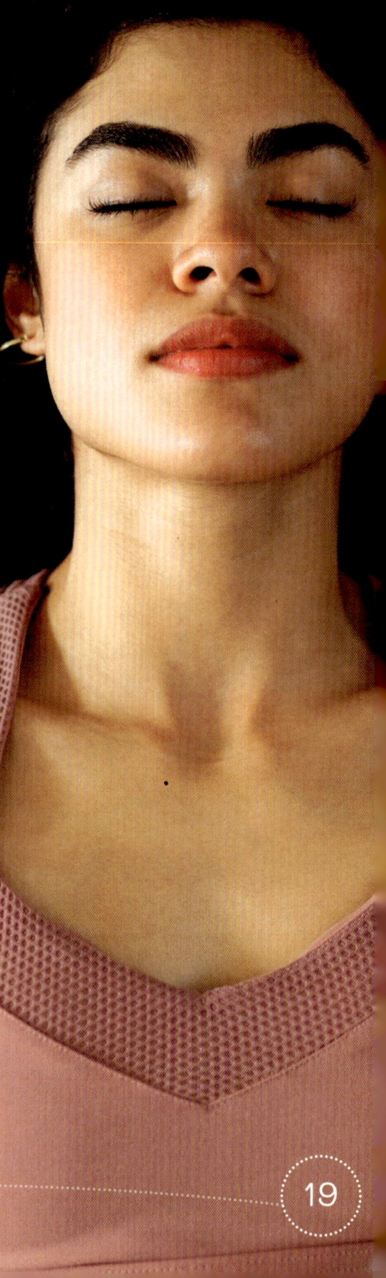

Slowly, the students start to move their bodies again. They carefully sit up and face the guru. Everyone puts their hands together in front of their chest. The guru says, "*Namaste*," and the class repeats it. *Namaste* means "I bow to you" in Sanskrit. It is often said at the end of yoga class to say thank you and to show respect for the other people in the class.

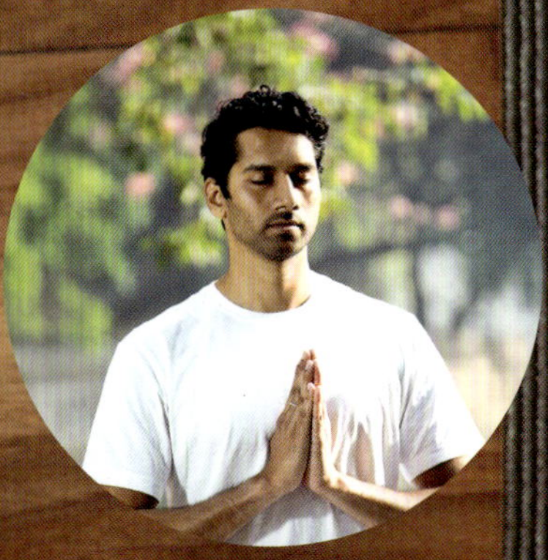

The Benefits of Yoga

Doing yoga has many benefits for the body and mind. Asanas make muscles stronger and more **flexible**. People that do yoga are able to move and balance more easily. They are more aware of their bodies and what they can do. This helps them with any other exercise they may do.

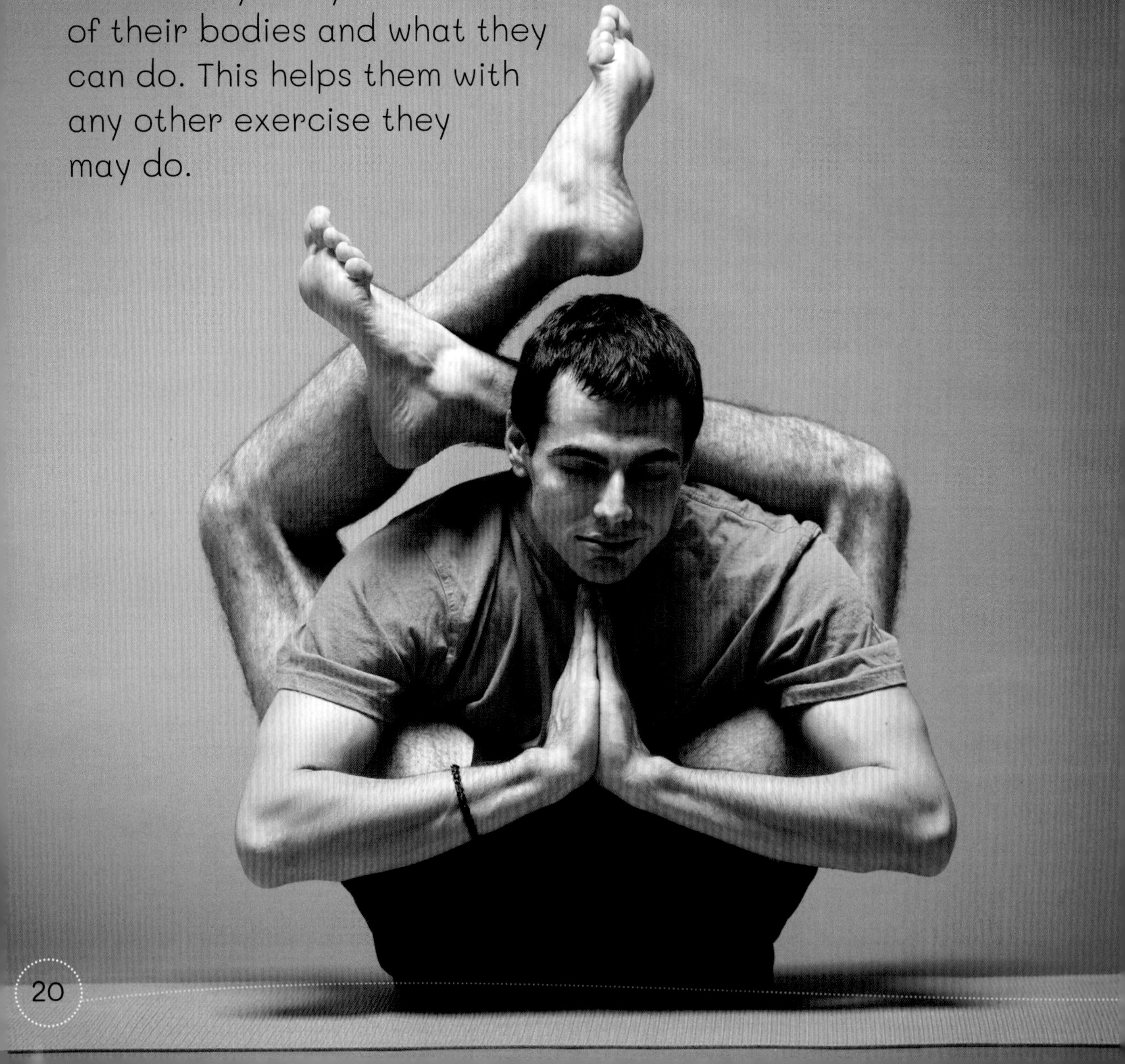

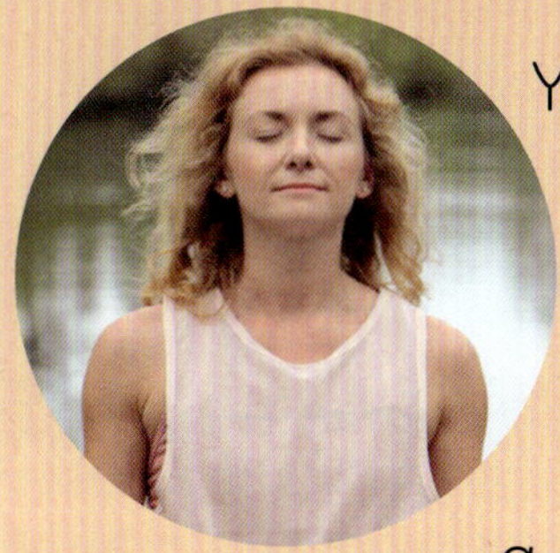

Yoga is also a good way to relieve stress. Stress causes the heart to pump faster, increasing blood pressure. This can lead to numerous health problems. Yoga calms the body, helping to lower a person's blood pressure. Pranayama techniques, in particular, can decrease stress and help people sleep better at night.

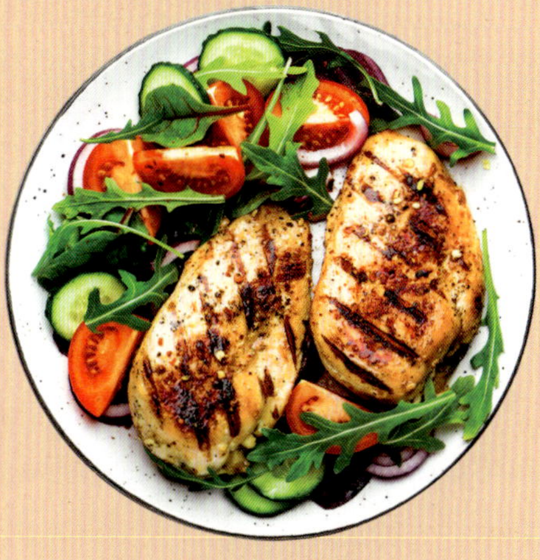

Yoga helps people live in the present moment and feel grateful for the things they have. Many yoga enthusiasts pay closer attention to what they eat, so they tend to eat healthier foods. People all over the world choose to practice yoga because it makes them feel happy and confident.

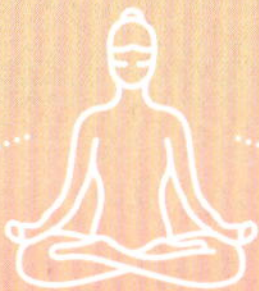

The **largest** yoga class in the world took place in Kota, Rajasthan, India, in **2018**, with **100,984** participants.

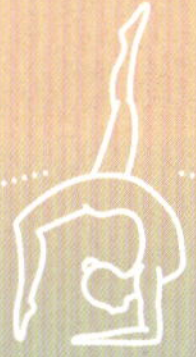

The Yoga Institute, in India, was started in **1918**. It was the **first** organized yoga center.

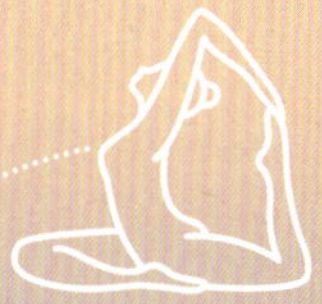

In 2012, Canadian Ida Herbert was named the **oldest** yoga teacher in the world. She was still teaching at **96 years of age**.

Yoga Quiz

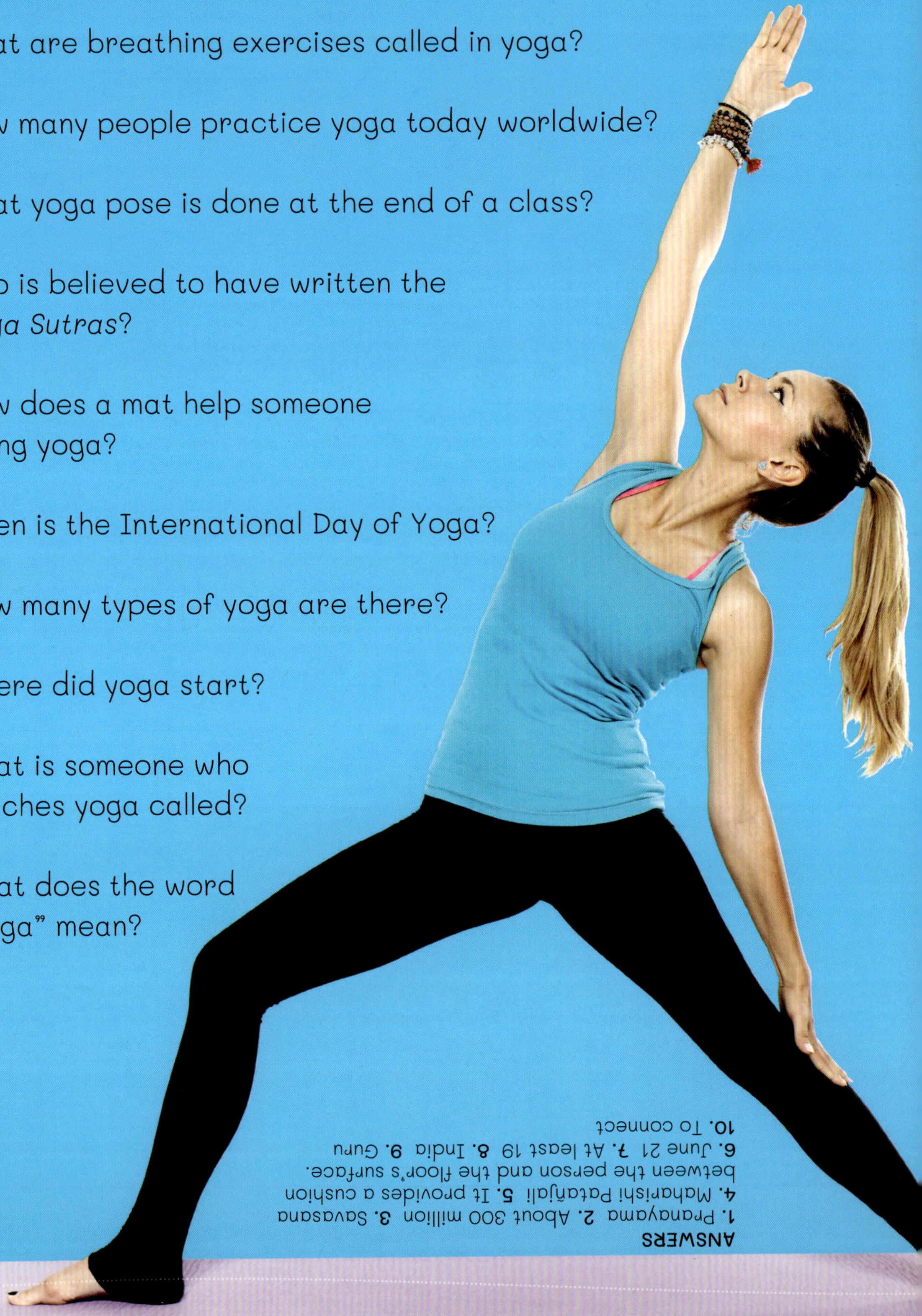

1. What are breathing exercises called in yoga?
2. How many people practice yoga today worldwide?
3. What yoga pose is done at the end of a class?
4. Who is believed to have written the *Yoga Sutras*?
5. How does a mat help someone doing yoga?
6. When is the International Day of Yoga?
7. How many types of yoga are there?
8. Where did yoga start?
9. What is someone who teaches yoga called?
10. What does the word "yoga" mean?

ANSWERS
1. Pranayama **2.** About 300 million **3.** Savasana
4. Maharishi Patañjali **5.** It provides a cushion between the person and the floor's surface.
6. June 21 **7.** At least 19 **8.** India **9.** Guru
10. To connect

Key Words

alignment: when the parts of the body are in the correct positions in relation to one another

flexible: able to bend without breaking

hydrated: having enough water

intention: the reason to do something; the desired outcome

meditation: mental exercises done for the purpose of reaching spiritual awareness

poses: specific positions in which a body is placed

practice: doing something regularly in a certain way

ratio: the relationship in quantity, amount, or size between two or more things

Sanskrit: an ancient language from India

stressed: in a state of mental or emotional strain

techniques: special ways of carrying out an activity

yogi: a person who has spent many years practicing yoga, and is considered to have reached an advanced level

Index

Get the best of both worlds.

AV2 bridges the gap between print and digital.

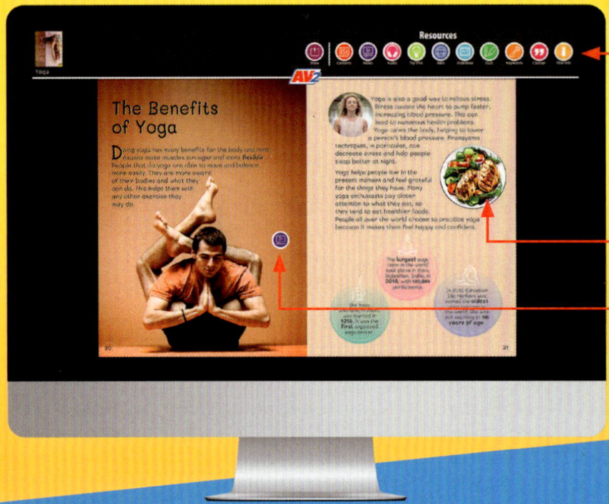

The expandable resources toolbar enables quick access to content including **videos**, **audio**, **activities**, **weblinks**, **slideshows**, **quizzes**, and **key words**.

Animated videos make static images come alive.

Resource icons on each page help readers to further **explore key concepts**.

Published by Lightbox Learning
276 5th Avenue, Suite 704 #917
New York, NY 10001
Website: www.openlightbox.com

Library of Congress Cataloging-in-Publication Data
Names: Noelle, Becky, author.
Title: Yoga / Becky Noelle.
Description: New York, NY : AV2, 2022. | Series: Wellness : mind body motion | Includes index. | Audience: Grades 2-3
Identifiers: LCCN 2021033657 (print) | LCCN 2021033658 (ebook) | ISBN 9781791142544 (library binding) | ISBN 9781791142551 (paperback) | ISBN 9781791142568
Subjects: LCSH: Hatha yoga for children--Juvenile literature. | Mindfulness (Psychology)--Juvenile literature.
Classification: LCC RJ133.7 .N64 2022 (print) | LCC RJ133.7 (ebook) | DDC 613.7/046083--dc23
LC record available at https://lccn.loc.gov/2021033657
LC ebook record available at https://lccn.loc.gov/2021033658

Printed in Guangzhou, China
1 2 3 4 5 6 7 8 9 0 25 24 23 22 21

092021
101120

Editor Heather Kissock
Designer Terry Paulhus

Photo Credits
Every reasonable effort has been made to trace ownership and to obtain permission to reprint copyright material. The publisher would be pleased to have any errors or omissions brought to its attention so that they may be corrected in subsequent printings. Lightbox Learning acknowledges Getty Images, Alamy, and Shutterstock as its primary photo suppliers for this title.